ISBN 978-1-998455-77-5 (Paperback)
ISBN 978-1-998455-78-2 (eBook)

Printed and bound in USA
Published by Loons Press

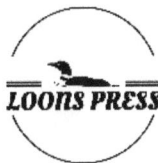

LOONS PRESS

I0096765

# Table Of Contents

# How To Reduce Liver Cancer Risk

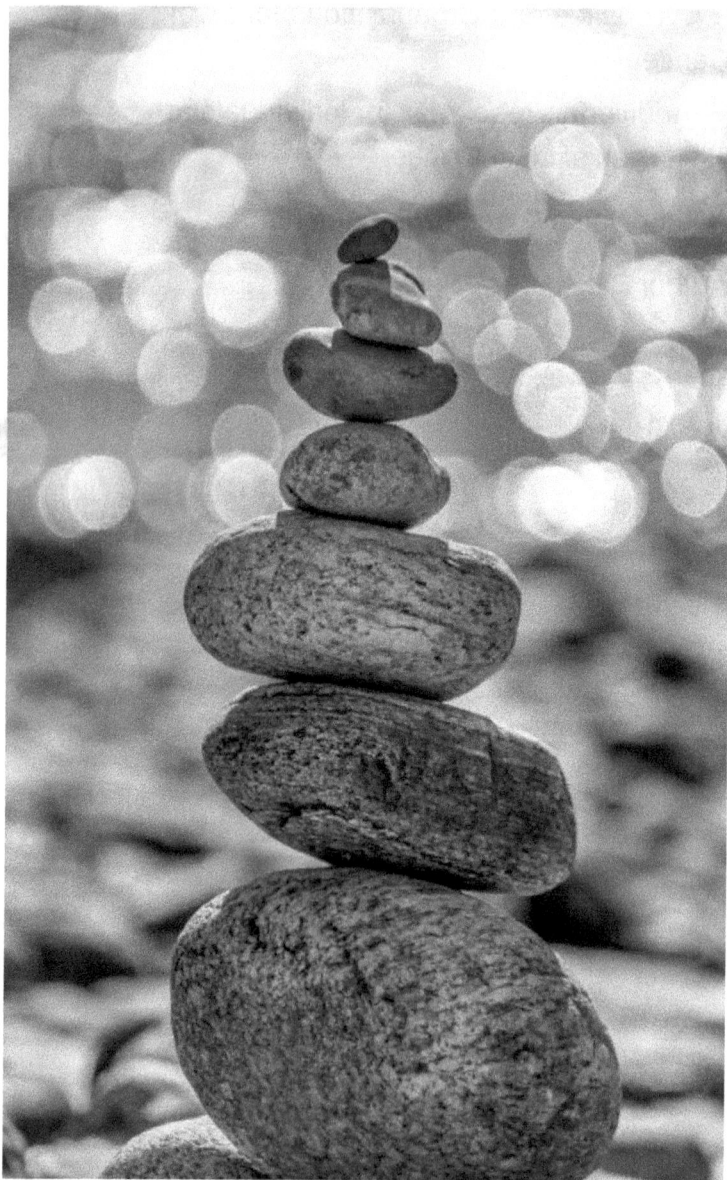

Tips and Strategies for Prevention

# Chapter 1

# Understanding Liver Cancer Risk Factors

## What is Liver Cancer?

Liver cancer is a serious and potentially life-threatening disease that occurs when abnormal cells in the liver grow out of control. The liver is a vital organ responsible for various functions, such as filtering toxins from the blood, producing bile, and storing energy. When cancer develops in the liver, it can interfere with these essential functions and lead to serious health complications.

There are several different types of liver cancer, with the most common being hepatocellular carcinoma (HCC). HCC typically develops in individuals with chronic liver diseases, such as hepatitis B or C, cirrhosis, or fatty liver disease. Other risk factors for liver cancer include excessive alcohol consumption, obesity, diabetes, and exposure to certain toxins or chemicals.

# How To Reduce Liver Cancer Risk

Early detection is crucial in the treatment of liver cancer, as the disease is often asymptomatic in its early stages. Symptoms of liver cancer may include abdominal pain, unexplained weight loss, jaundice, and fatigue.

If you are at risk for liver cancer due to underlying liver disease or other risk factors, it is important to undergo regular screenings and diagnostic tests to detect any abnormalities early on.

There are several strategies you can implement to lower your risk of developing liver cancer. First and foremost, maintaining a healthy lifestyle is key. This includes eating a balanced diet, exercising regularly, avoiding excessive alcohol consumption, and not smoking.

Additionally, individuals at risk for liver cancer should undergo regular screenings and vaccinations for hepatitis B and C, as these viruses are major risk factors for liver cancer.

In conclusion, liver cancer is a serious and potentially deadly disease that can be prevented with early detection and lifestyle modifications. By understanding the risk factors for liver cancer and implementing preventive strategies, individuals can lower their risk of developing this devastating disease.

It is important for those at risk for liver cancer to stay informed, undergo regular screenings, and work closely with their healthcare providers to monitor and manage their liver health.

## Common Risk Factors for Liver Cancer

Liver cancer is a serious and potentially life-threatening condition that can be caused by a variety of risk factors. Understanding these risk factors is essential for individuals who are concerned about their liver cancer risk. By being aware of common risk factors, individuals can take proactive steps to reduce their risk and protect their liver health.

One common risk factor for liver cancer is chronic infection with hepatitis B or hepatitis C virus. These viruses can cause inflammation and damage to the liver over time, increasing the risk of developing liver cancer. Individuals who have been diagnosed with hepatitis B or hepatitis C should work closely with their healthcare provider to manage their condition and reduce their risk of liver cancer.

Another important risk factor for liver cancer is excessive alcohol consumption. Chronic alcohol abuse can lead to liver damage and cirrhosis, which are both risk factors for liver cancer. Individuals who consume alcohol should do so in moderation and seek help if they are struggling to control their drinking habits. By reducing alcohol consumption, individuals can lower their risk of developing liver cancer.

Obesity and non-alcoholic fatty liver disease are also common risk factors for liver cancer. Excess body weight and fat accumulation in the liver can lead to inflammation and scarring, increasing the risk of liver cancer.

Individuals who are overweight or have been diagnosed with fatty liver disease should focus on maintaining a healthy weight through diet and exercise to reduce their risk of liver cancer.

Certain genetic factors can also increase an individual's risk of developing liver cancer. Individuals with a family history of liver cancer or certain genetic conditions, such as hemochromatosis or alpha-1 antitrypsin deficiency, may be at higher risk. It is important for individuals with these genetic risk factors to work closely with their healthcare provider to monitor their liver health and take steps to reduce their risk of liver cancer.

Overall, understanding common risk factors for liver cancer is essential for individuals who are concerned about their liver health. By taking proactive steps to reduce these risk factors, individuals can lower their risk of developing liver cancer and protect their overall health. Working with healthcare providers to manage chronic conditions, maintain a healthy weight, and make positive lifestyle choices can all help individuals reduce their risk of liver cancer and live healthier, longer lives.

## Genetic Factors that Increase Liver Cancer Risk

Liver cancer is a serious disease that can have devastating consequences for those who are affected by it. While there are many factors that can contribute to an increased risk of developing liver cancer, one of the most important is genetics. Genetic factors play a significant role in determining an individual's susceptibility to liver cancer, and understanding these factors can help people take steps to reduce their risk.

One of the most well-known genetic factors that can increase the risk of liver cancer is a family history of the disease. If you have a close relative who has been diagnosed with liver cancer, you may be at an increased risk of developing the disease yourself. This is because certain genetic mutations that increase the risk of liver cancer can be passed down from one generation to the next.

If you have a family history of liver cancer, it is important to talk to your healthcare provider about your risk and discuss ways to reduce it.

In addition to family history, certain genetic conditions can also increase the risk of liver cancer. For example, individuals with hereditary hemochromatosis, a condition that causes the body to absorb too much iron, are at an increased risk of developing liver cancer.

Similarly, individuals with certain genetic mutations, such as those associated with Lynch syndrome, may also have a higher risk of developing liver cancer. If you have one of these genetic conditions, it is important to work closely with your healthcare provider to monitor your liver health and take steps to reduce your risk of developing liver cancer.

Another important genetic factor that can increase the risk of liver cancer is the presence of certain viral infections. Chronic infections with hepatitis B or hepatitis C viruses can lead to liver inflammation and damage, which can increase the risk of developing liver cancer. These viral infections can be passed down from parent to child or acquired through contact with infected blood or bodily fluids.

# How To Reduce Liver Cancer Risk

If you have a history of hepatitis B or hepatitis C infection, it is important to work with your healthcare provider to monitor your liver health and take steps to reduce your risk of developing liver cancer.

Overall, genetic factors play a significant role in determining an individual's risk of developing liver cancer. If you have a family history of the disease, a genetic condition that increases the risk of liver cancer, or a history of viral infections that can damage the liver, it is important to work closely with your healthcare provider to monitor your liver health and take steps to reduce your risk.

By understanding the genetic factors that can increase the risk of liver cancer and taking proactive steps to address them, individuals can reduce their risk of developing this serious disease.

## Lifestyle Choices and Liver Cancer Risk

Lifestyle choices play a significant role in determining an individual's risk of developing liver cancer. By making conscious decisions about diet, exercise, and other habits, you can greatly reduce your chances of developing this deadly disease.

In this subchapter, we will explore the various lifestyle choices that can impact your liver cancer risk and provide practical tips and strategies for prevention.

One of the most important lifestyle choices that can affect your risk of liver cancer is your diet. Consuming a diet high in processed foods, saturated fats, and sugar can increase inflammation in the body and put extra strain on the liver. Instead, focus on eating a balanced diet rich in fruits, vegetables, whole grains, and lean proteins. These foods provide essential nutrients that support liver health and reduce the risk of developing cancer.

Regular exercise is another key factor in reducing your risk of liver cancer. Physical activity helps to maintain a healthy weight, improve circulation, and support overall liver function. Aim for at least 30 minutes of moderate exercise most days of the week to reap the benefits of a healthy lifestyle.

Whether you prefer walking, cycling, dancing, or yoga, find an activity that you enjoy and make it a regular part of your routine.

Avoiding harmful habits such as smoking and excessive alcohol consumption is also crucial for lowering your liver cancer risk. Both smoking and heavy drinking can damage liver cells and increase the likelihood of developing cancer.

If you currently smoke or drink excessively, seek support to help you quit these habits and protect your liver health. Making these changes may be challenging, but the long-term benefits for your health are well worth the effort.

In conclusion, your lifestyle choices have a significant impact on your risk of developing liver cancer. By adopting a healthy diet, staying physically active, and avoiding harmful habits, you can greatly reduce your chances of developing this deadly disease. Take control of your health and make positive changes today to protect your liver and lower your cancer risk. Remember, prevention is key when it comes to maintaining a healthy lifestyle and reducing your risk of liver cancer.

# How To Reduce Liver Cancer Risk

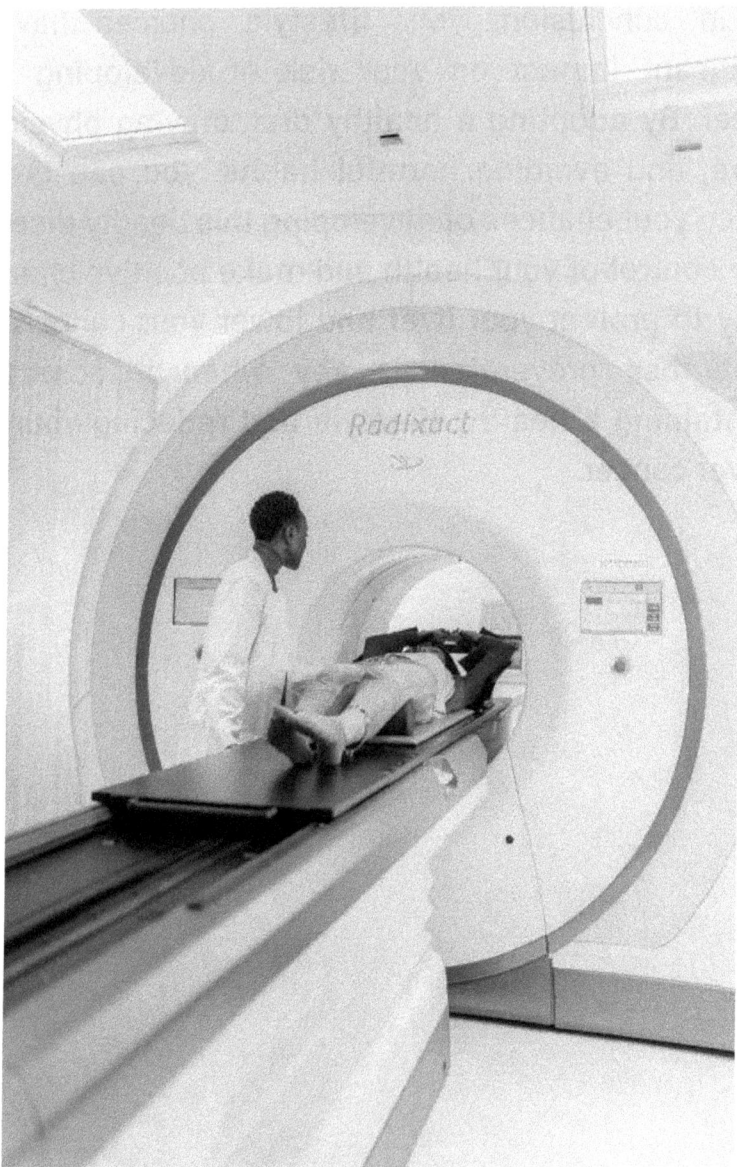

# Chapter 2

# Importance of Early Detection and Diagnosis

## Signs and Symptoms of Liver Cancer

Liver cancer is a serious condition that can have devastating effects on one's health and well-being. Understanding the signs and symptoms of liver cancer is crucial in order to catch the disease early and increase the chances of successful treatment.

Some common signs of liver cancer include unexplained weight loss, loss of appetite, and feeling full even after eating only a small amount of food. These symptoms can be indicative of a tumor in the liver that is affecting the body's ability to process nutrients properly.

Another common symptom of liver cancer is jaundice, which is a condition that causes the skin and eyes to appear yellow. Jaundice occurs when the liver is unable to properly process bilirubin, a waste product that is normally excreted in bile. When the liver is not functioning properly, bilirubin can build up in the blood and cause the characteristic yellowing of the skin and eyes. Jaundice is a serious symptom that should be evaluated by a healthcare provider as soon as possible.

In addition to jaundice, other symptoms of liver cancer can include abdominal pain, swelling in the abdomen, and a feeling of fullness or bloating. These symptoms can be caused by the pressure of a tumor on the liver or surrounding organs, as well as the accumulation of fluid in the abdomen, a condition known as ascites.

It is important to pay attention to any changes in your body and seek medical attention if you experience any of these symptoms.

Some people with liver cancer may also experience nausea, vomiting, and fatigue. These symptoms can be caused by the body's inability to properly process toxins and waste products, as well as the strain that the disease puts on the body's energy reserves.

If you are experiencing persistent nausea, vomiting, or fatigue, it is important to discuss these symptoms with your healthcare provider to determine the underlying cause.

Overall, being aware of the signs and symptoms of liver cancer is crucial for anyone who is at risk for the disease. By recognizing these symptoms early and seeking medical attention promptly, individuals can increase their chances of successful treatment and improve their overall prognosis.

If you are concerned about your risk of liver cancer or are experiencing any of the symptoms mentioned here, it is important to speak with your healthcare provider to discuss your concerns and develop a plan for monitoring and managing your risk.

## Diagnostic Tests for Liver Cancer

In order to effectively reduce your risk of developing liver cancer, it is important to understand the diagnostic tests available for early detection. These tests can help identify any abnormalities in the liver at an early stage, allowing for prompt treatment and improved outcomes.

Here, we will discuss some of the key diagnostic tests for liver cancer that you should be aware of.

One of the most common diagnostic tests for liver cancer is a liver function test. This test measures the levels of certain enzymes and proteins in the blood that are produced by the liver. Abnormal levels of these substances can indicate liver damage or dysfunction, which may be a sign of liver cancer.

Your doctor may recommend this test if you are at risk for liver cancer or if you are experiencing symptoms such as jaundice, abdominal pain, or unexplained weight loss.

Imaging tests such as ultrasound, CT scans, and MRI scans can also be used to diagnose liver cancer. These tests allow doctors to visualize the liver and identify any abnormalities, such as tumors or lesions. Imaging tests can help determine the size and location of a tumor, as well as whether it has spread to other parts of the body. If a suspicious mass is detected, your doctor may recommend further testing, such as a biopsy, to confirm a diagnosis of liver cancer.

A biopsy is a procedure in which a small sample of tissue is taken from the liver and examined under a microscope. This test is the most definitive way to diagnose liver cancer, as it allows doctors to analyze the cells for signs of cancer.

A biopsy can also help determine the type and stage of liver cancer, which is important for developing an appropriate treatment plan. Your doctor may recommend a biopsy if other tests suggest the presence of liver cancer or if you are at high risk for the disease.

In addition to these diagnostic tests, your doctor may also recommend screening tests for liver cancer if you are at increased risk. These tests are typically recommended for individuals with a family history of liver cancer, a history of liver disease, or other risk factors such as heavy alcohol use or obesity. Screening tests can help detect liver cancer at an early stage, when it is most treatable. By staying informed about the diagnostic tests available for liver cancer and working closely with your healthcare provider, you can take proactive steps to reduce your risk of developing this devastating disease.

## The Role of Screening in Lowering Liver Cancer Risk

Early detection is key to lowering the risk of developing liver cancer. Screening plays a crucial role in identifying potential issues before they progress to more serious stages. For people who have a higher risk of liver cancer, such as those with a history of hepatitis B or C, cirrhosis, or a family history of liver cancer, regular screening can help catch any abnormalities early on.

# How To Reduce Liver Cancer Risk

By detecting liver cancer at an early stage, treatment options are more effective, and the chances of successful outcomes are higher.

Screening for liver cancer typically involves a combination of imaging tests, such as ultrasounds, CT scans, or MRIs, and blood tests to check for specific markers that may indicate the presence of liver cancer. These screening methods are non-invasive and relatively quick, making them accessible to a wide range of individuals. By undergoing regular screenings as recommended by healthcare professionals, individuals can stay proactive in monitoring their liver health and catching any potential issues early.

In addition to regular screening, maintaining a healthy lifestyle plays a significant role in lowering liver cancer risk. Eating a balanced diet, exercising regularly, and avoiding excessive alcohol consumption are all essential factors in keeping the liver healthy. By taking care of the liver through lifestyle choices, individuals can reduce their overall risk of developing liver cancer and other liver-related conditions. Screening is just one part of a comprehensive approach to lowering liver cancer risk.

For those at higher risk of liver cancer, such as individuals with chronic liver conditions or a family history of the disease, it is especially important to stay vigilant about screening. Regular check-ups with healthcare providers and following recommended screening guidelines can help catch any potential issues early on.

By being proactive about monitoring liver health and staying informed about the latest screening methods, individuals can take control of their health and reduce their risk of developing liver cancer.

In conclusion, screening plays a crucial role in lowering liver cancer risk by detecting potential issues early on and allowing for timely intervention. By combining regular screenings with a healthy lifestyle, individuals can take proactive steps towards reducing their risk of developing liver cancer. Staying informed about screening guidelines and working closely with healthcare providers can help individuals stay on top of their liver health and make informed decisions about their care.

By taking a comprehensive approach to lowering liver cancer risk, individuals can empower themselves to lead healthier lives and reduce their risk of developing this serious disease.

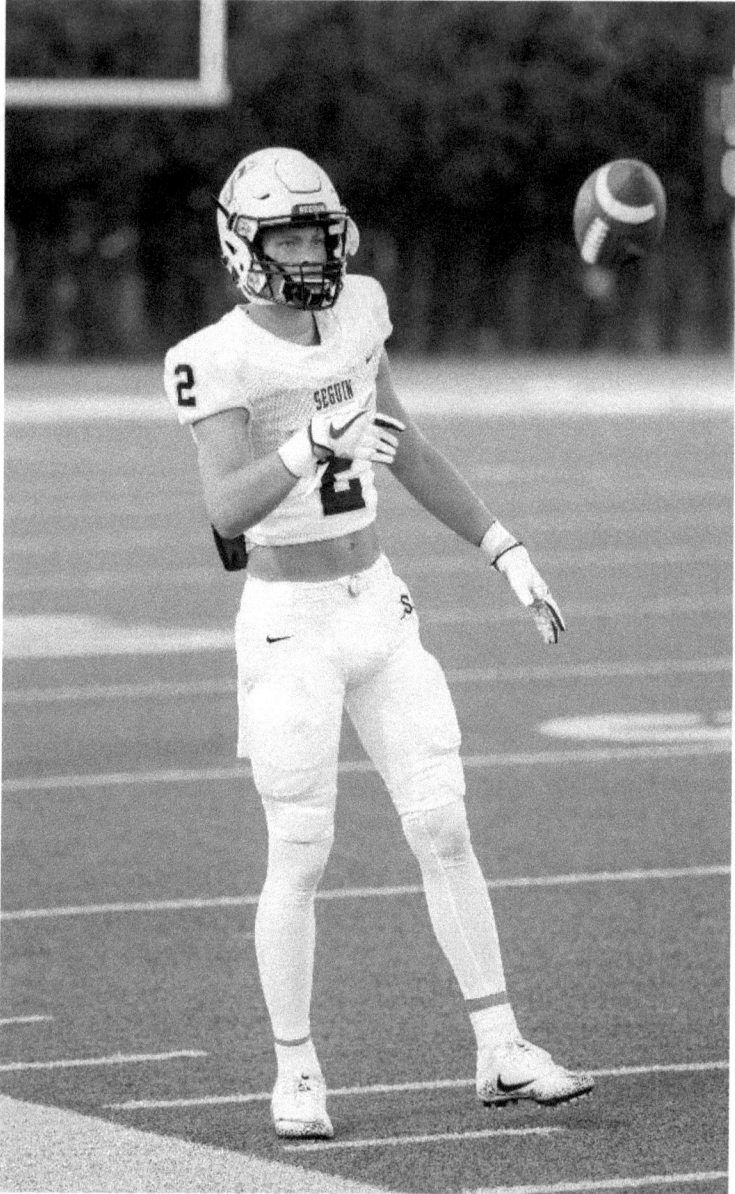

# Chapter 3

# Healthy Habits for Lowering Liver Cancer Risk

## Maintaining a Healthy Weight

Maintaining a healthy weight is an important factor in reducing your risk of liver cancer. Obesity is a known risk factor for liver cancer, as excess fat can lead to inflammation and scarring of the liver, which can increase your chances of developing cancer. By maintaining a healthy weight, you can reduce the strain on your liver and lower your risk of developing liver cancer.

One way to maintain a healthy weight is to eat a balanced diet that is rich in fruits, vegetables, whole grains, and lean proteins. Avoiding processed foods, sugary drinks, and high-fat foods can help you maintain a healthy weight and reduce your risk of liver cancer. It is also important to watch your portion sizes and avoid overeating, as consuming too many calories can lead to weight gain and increase your risk of developing liver cancer.

In addition to eating a healthy diet, regular exercise is also important for maintaining a healthy weight and reducing your risk of liver cancer. Exercise can help you burn calories, build muscle, and improve your overall health. Aim for at least 150 minutes of moderate-intensity exercise each week, such as brisk walking, cycling, or swimming.

By incorporating regular exercise into your routine, you can help maintain a healthy weight and lower your risk of developing liver cancer.

It is also important to monitor your weight regularly and make adjustments to your diet and exercise routine as needed. If you notice that you are gaining weight, try increasing your physical activity or cutting back on high-calorie foods.

By staying mindful of your weight and taking proactive steps to maintain a healthy weight, you can reduce your risk of liver cancer and improve your overall health.

In conclusion, maintaining a healthy weight is an essential part of reducing your risk of liver cancer. By eating a balanced diet, engaging in regular exercise, and monitoring your weight, you can help protect your liver and lower your chances of developing cancer.

Remember to consult with your healthcare provider for personalized recommendations on how to maintain a healthy weight and reduce your risk of liver cancer.

## Eating a Balanced Diet

Eating a balanced diet is crucial for reducing your risk of developing liver cancer. A diet that is high in fruits, vegetables, whole grains, and lean proteins can help to support a healthy liver and overall well-being.

By incorporating a variety of nutrient-rich foods into your meals, you can provide your body with the essential vitamins and minerals it needs to function optimally and reduce your risk of developing liver cancer.

One key component of a balanced diet is limiting your intake of processed foods, sugary drinks, and foods high in saturated fats. These types of foods can contribute to inflammation in the body and put added stress on the liver, increasing your risk of developing liver cancer. By focusing on whole, unprocessed foods, you can help to support liver health and reduce your risk of cancer.

In addition to eating a variety of nutrient-rich foods, it is important to stay hydrated and limit your intake of alcohol. Drinking plenty of water throughout the day can help to flush toxins from the body and support liver function. Limiting alcohol consumption is also important, as excessive alcohol intake can cause damage to the liver and increase your risk of developing liver cancer.

Another important aspect of eating a balanced diet is maintaining a healthy weight. Being overweight or obese can increase your risk of developing liver cancer, as excess body fat can lead to inflammation and damage to the liver.

By eating a balanced diet and engaging in regular physical activity, you can help to maintain a healthy weight and reduce your risk of developing liver cancer.

In conclusion, eating a balanced diet is essential for reducing your risk of developing liver cancer. By focusing on nutrient-rich foods, limiting processed foods and sugary drinks, staying hydrated, and maintaining a healthy weight, you can support liver health and reduce your risk of cancer. Making small changes to your diet and lifestyle can have a significant impact on your overall health and well-being, helping to lower your risk of developing liver cancer.

## Limiting Alcohol Consumption

Limiting alcohol consumption is crucial for individuals who have a liver cancer risk, as excessive alcohol consumption can significantly increase the likelihood of developing liver cancer. Alcohol is processed by the liver, and over time, heavy drinking can lead to inflammation and scarring of the liver, known as cirrhosis.

This damage increases the risk of developing liver cancer, making it essential to limit alcohol intake to reduce this risk.

One of the most effective ways to limit alcohol consumption is to set a daily or weekly limit for yourself. The recommended limit for men is no more than two drinks per day, while for women, it is no more than one drink per day. By setting a limit and sticking to it, you can reduce the strain on your liver and decrease your risk of developing liver cancer.

It is also important to be mindful of the size of your drinks, as many alcoholic beverages contain more than one standard drink. Be sure to measure your drinks and keep track of how many standard drinks you are consuming to ensure that you are staying within your limit.

Additionally, consider opting for non-alcoholic or low-alcohol alternatives when socializing or relaxing, as this can help reduce your overall alcohol intake.

If you find it challenging to limit your alcohol consumption on your own, consider seeking support from friends, family, or a healthcare professional. They can provide encouragement, accountability, and resources to help you cut back on your drinking.

Additionally, joining a support group or seeking therapy can be beneficial for individuals struggling with alcohol use disorder, as they can provide guidance and strategies for reducing alcohol consumption.

By taking steps to limit alcohol consumption, individuals with a liver cancer risk can significantly reduce their chances of developing this deadly disease. Making small changes to your drinking habits can have a big impact on your liver health and overall well-being.

Remember, moderation is key when it comes to alcohol consumption, and by setting limits and seeking support when needed, you can lower your liver cancer risk and improve your overall health.

## Exercising Regularly

Exercising regularly is one of the most effective ways to reduce your risk of developing liver cancer. Physical activity has been shown to help lower inflammation in the body, which can reduce the risk of developing cancerous cells in the liver.

By incorporating regular exercise into your routine, you can improve your overall health and significantly lower your chances of developing liver cancer.

One of the key benefits of regular exercise is its ability to help control your weight. Being overweight or obese is a major risk factor for liver cancer, so maintaining a healthy weight through regular physical activity can significantly reduce your risk. Exercise helps to burn calories and build muscle, which can help you achieve and maintain a healthy weight.

By engaging in regular exercise, you can lower your risk of developing liver cancer and improve your overall health.

In addition to helping control weight, regular exercise can also help improve the function of your liver. Exercise has been shown to help reduce the build-up of fat in the liver, which can lead to liver damage and increase the risk of developing liver cancer.

By engaging in physical activity on a regular basis, you can help keep your liver healthy and reduce your risk of developing liver cancer.

Furthermore, regular exercise has been shown to boost the immune system, which plays a crucial role in fighting off cancer cells. By engaging in physical activity, you can strengthen your immune system and improve its ability to detect and destroy cancerous cells in the body. This can help reduce your risk of developing liver cancer and improve your overall health and well-being.

# How To Reduce Liver Cancer Risk

Overall, incorporating regular exercise into your routine is an essential strategy for reducing your risk of developing liver cancer. By maintaining a healthy weight, improving liver function, and boosting your immune system through physical activity, you can significantly lower your chances of developing this deadly disease. Make exercise a priority in your daily life to protect your liver health and reduce your risk of liver cancer.

# How To Reduce Liver Cancer Risk

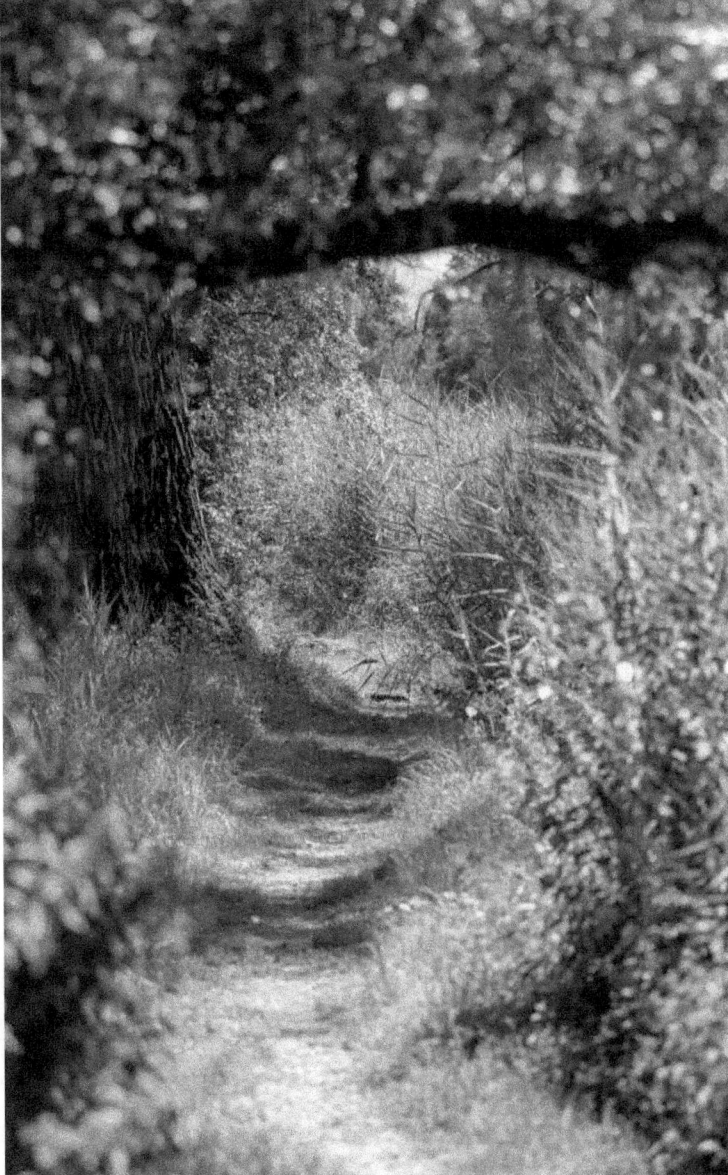

# Chapter 4

# Avoiding Known Liver Cancer Risk Factors

## Hepatitis B and C Prevention

Hepatitis B and C are two of the leading causes of liver cancer worldwide. In order to lower your risk of developing liver cancer, it is crucial to take steps to prevent these viral infections. Hepatitis B and C are spread through contact with infected blood or body fluids, so it is important to practice safe sex, avoid sharing needles or other drug paraphernalia, and ensure that any tattoos or piercings are done with sterile equipment.

One of the most effective ways to prevent hepatitis B is through vaccination. The hepatitis B vaccine is safe, effective, and widely available. It is recommended for all infants, as well as for adults who are at increased risk of infection, such as healthcare workers, people with multiple sexual partners, and individuals who inject drugs.

By getting vaccinated against hepatitis B, you can greatly reduce your risk of developing liver cancer.

In addition to vaccination, it is important to practice good hygiene to prevent the spread of hepatitis B and C. This includes washing your hands frequently, especially after using the bathroom or coming into contact with blood or body fluids. It is also important to avoid sharing personal items such as toothbrushes or razors, which can potentially transmit the viruses. By practicing good hygiene, you can lower your risk of contracting hepatitis B and C and reduce your overall risk of developing liver cancer.

For individuals who are already infected with hepatitis B or C, it is important to seek proper medical care and follow your healthcare provider's recommendations for treatment. Antiviral medications can help to manage the viruses and reduce the risk of liver damage and cancer. It is also important to avoid alcohol and maintain a healthy lifestyle, including eating a balanced diet and getting regular exercise. By taking these steps, you can help to lower your risk of developing liver cancer and improve your overall health and well-being.

In conclusion, preventing hepatitis B and C is key to lowering your risk of developing liver cancer. By getting vaccinated, practicing good hygiene, seeking proper medical care if infected, and maintaining a healthy lifestyle, you can reduce your risk of liver cancer and improve your overall health.

Remember that prevention is always better than treatment, so take steps now to protect yourself from these viral infections and lower your risk of liver cancer.

## Avoiding Exposure to Toxins and Chemicals

Avoiding exposure to toxins and chemicals is a crucial step in lowering your risk of developing liver cancer. Many toxins and chemicals can be harmful to your liver, putting you at an increased risk for developing this type of cancer. By taking proactive measures to reduce your exposure to these harmful substances, you can protect your liver and decrease your chances of developing liver cancer.

# How To Reduce Liver Cancer Risk

One of the most important ways to avoid exposure to toxins and chemicals is to be mindful of what you are putting into your body. This includes being cautious of the food and drinks you consume, as well as the medications and supplements you take. Try to choose organic and natural products whenever possible, and avoid processed foods that may contain harmful chemicals and additives.

Additionally, be sure to follow proper dosing instructions for medications and supplements to minimize any potential harm to your liver.

In addition to being mindful of what you are putting into your body, it is also important to be aware of your environment and the potential toxins and chemicals that may be present. If you work in an industry where you may be exposed to harmful substances, be sure to take proper precautions and follow safety guidelines to protect yourself. This may include wearing protective gear, such as gloves and masks, and following proper ventilation protocols to minimize exposure to harmful fumes and chemicals.

Another important aspect of avoiding exposure to toxins and chemicals is to be mindful of the products you use in your home and personal care routine. Many household cleaners, beauty products, and other items contain harmful chemicals that can be absorbed through your skin or inhaled, putting added stress on your liver.

Consider switching to natural and eco-friendly alternatives to reduce your exposure to harmful toxins and chemicals in your home.

By taking proactive steps to avoid exposure to toxins and chemicals, you can significantly lower your risk of developing liver cancer. Remember to be mindful of what you are putting into your body, be aware of your environment, and choose natural and eco-friendly products whenever possible.

By prioritizing your liver health and reducing your exposure to harmful substances, you can protect yourself and decrease your risk of developing liver cancer.

## Managing Diabetes and Other Chronic Conditions

Managing diabetes and other chronic conditions is crucial for reducing your risk of developing liver cancer. Diabetes is a known risk factor for liver cancer, as it can lead to inflammation and scarring of the liver, increasing the likelihood of cancerous growths.

By effectively managing your diabetes through medication, diet, and exercise, you can lower your risk of developing liver cancer.

In addition to diabetes, other chronic conditions such as obesity, high blood pressure, and high cholesterol can also increase your risk of liver cancer. It is important to work with your healthcare provider to effectively manage these conditions through lifestyle changes, medication, and regular monitoring. By keeping these conditions under control, you can reduce your overall risk of developing liver cancer.

# How To Reduce Liver Cancer Risk

A key component of managing diabetes and other chronic conditions is maintaining a healthy lifestyle. This includes eating a balanced diet rich in fruits, vegetables, whole grains, and lean proteins, as well as engaging in regular physical activity. By making healthy choices and staying active, you can not only improve your overall health but also reduce your risk of liver cancer.

Regular monitoring and screening are also important for managing diabetes and other chronic conditions. By keeping track of your blood sugar levels, blood pressure, cholesterol levels, and weight, you can identify any changes or potential issues early on. This allows your doctors to make necessary adjustments to your treatment plan and reduce your risk of complications, including liver cancer.

In conclusion, managing diabetes and other chronic conditions is essential for reducing your risk of liver cancer. By working with your healthcare provider to effectively manage these conditions through medication, diet, exercise, and regular monitoring, you can take control of your health and lower your risk of developing liver cancer.

Remember that prevention is key, and by making healthy choices and staying proactive about your health, you can reduce your liver cancer risk and live a longer, healthier life.

# How To Reduce Liver Cancer Risk

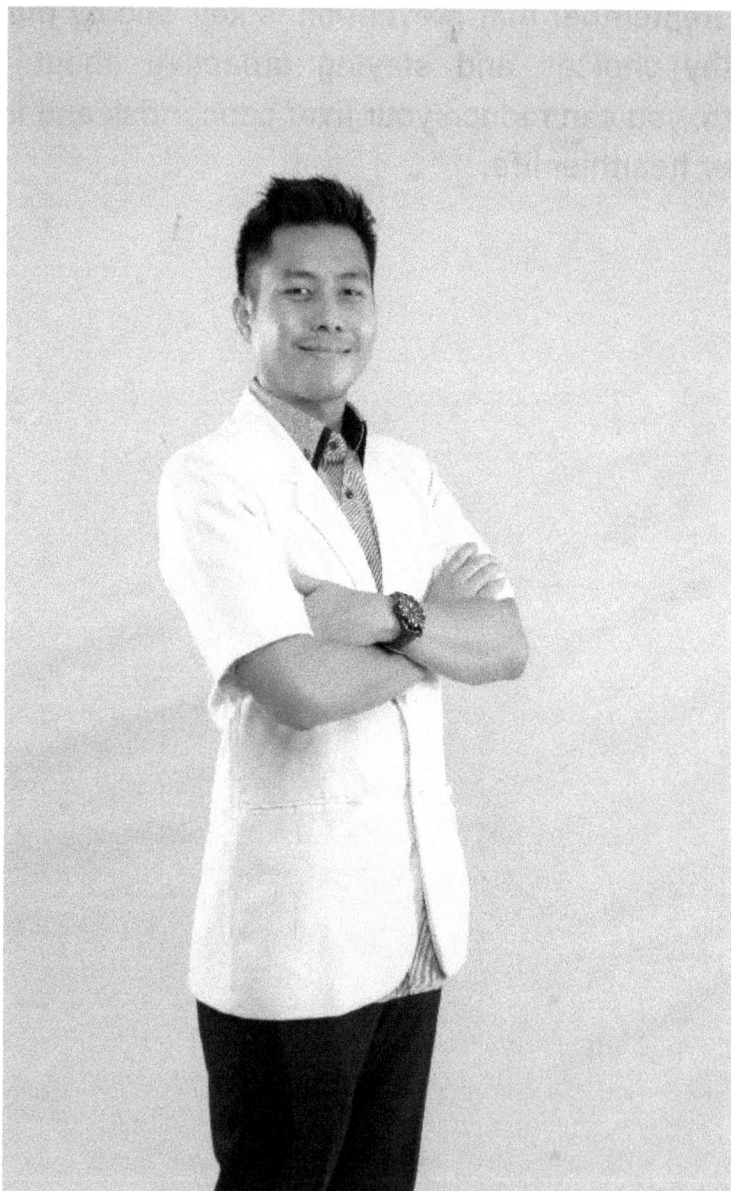

# Chapter 5

# Seeking Support and Resources for Liver Cancer Prevention

## Connecting with Healthcare Providers

Connecting with healthcare providers is a crucial step in managing and reducing your risk of liver cancer. Your healthcare team can provide you with important information, guidance, and resources to help you make informed decisions about your health.

When meeting with your healthcare provider, be sure to discuss your personal and family medical history, as well as any lifestyle factors that may increase your risk of liver cancer. This information can help your provider assess your risk level and develop a personalized plan for prevention.

# How To Reduce Liver Cancer Risk

It is important to establish open and honest communication with your healthcare providers. Be sure to ask questions, express any concerns you may have, and seek clarification on any information or recommendations provided to you. Remember, your healthcare team is there to support you and help you make the best choices for your health.

In addition to regular check-ups and screenings, your healthcare provider may recommend certain lifestyle changes to help lower your risk of liver cancer. These may include maintaining a healthy weight, eating a balanced diet, exercising regularly, limiting alcohol consumption, and avoiding exposure to toxins such as tobacco and certain chemicals.

By working closely with your healthcare providers and following their recommendations, you can take proactive steps to lower your risk of liver cancer. Remember, early detection and prevention are key in managing this disease, so be sure to stay informed, engaged, and proactive in your healthcare journey.

## Joining Support Groups for Liver Cancer Prevention

Joining support groups for liver cancer prevention can be a valuable resource for individuals who are at risk of developing the disease. These groups provide a safe space for individuals to share their experiences, fears, and concerns with others who are facing similar challenges.

By connecting with others who are also at risk of developing liver cancer, individuals can gain valuable insights and support to help them navigate their own health journey.

Support groups for liver cancer prevention can also provide individuals with access to valuable information and resources. Through these groups, individuals can learn about the latest research and developments in liver cancer prevention, as well as discover new strategies and tips for reducing their risk of developing the disease. This information can be empowering and motivating, helping individuals to take proactive steps towards protecting their liver health.

In addition to providing information and support, joining a support group for liver cancer prevention can also help individuals to feel less alone in their journey. Liver cancer can be a challenging and isolating experience, but connecting with others who understand what you are going through can provide a sense of community and solidarity.

By sharing your story and listening to the experiences of others, you can gain a sense of perspective and hope that can be invaluable in navigating your own health challenges.

Support groups for liver cancer prevention can also provide practical tips and strategies for reducing your risk of developing the disease. From dietary recommendations to lifestyle changes, support groups can offer valuable insights and guidance on how to make healthier choices that can protect your liver health. By connecting with others who are also focused on prevention, you can gain motivation and inspiration to make positive changes in your own life.

In conclusion, joining a support group for liver cancer prevention can be a valuable resource for individuals who are at risk of developing the disease. These groups provide a safe space for individuals to share their experiences, gain access to valuable information and resources, feel less alone in their journey, and receive practical tips and strategies for reducing their risk of developing liver cancer. By connecting with others who understand what you are going through, you can gain the support and motivation you need to take proactive steps towards protecting your liver health.

## Utilizing Online Resources for Liver Cancer Prevention

In today's digital age, there is a wealth of information available at our fingertips that can help us reduce our risk of developing liver cancer. Online resources provide a convenient and accessible way to educate ourselves on the steps we can take to prevent this deadly disease. By utilizing these resources, individuals who have a higher risk of developing liver cancer can empower themselves with knowledge and tools to lower their risk.

# How To Reduce Liver Cancer Risk

One of the most valuable online resources for liver cancer prevention is reputable medical websites and organizations. These websites offer comprehensive information on the risk factors for liver cancer, as well as tips and strategies for prevention. By visiting these websites, individuals can learn about the importance of maintaining a healthy lifestyle, including eating a balanced diet, exercising regularly, and avoiding excessive alcohol consumption. These resources also provide information on the importance of regular screenings and vaccinations for hepatitis B and C, which are major risk factors for liver cancer.

Another valuable online resource for liver cancer prevention is online support groups and forums. These platforms provide individuals with the opportunity to connect with others who are at a higher risk of developing liver cancer. By sharing experiences, tips, and strategies for prevention, individuals can learn from each other and feel supported in their efforts to reduce their risk. Online support groups can also provide a sense of community and belonging, which can be invaluable for individuals facing the challenges of liver cancer risk.

Social media platforms are also a valuable tool for liver cancer prevention. Many organizations and individuals dedicated to raising awareness about liver cancer prevention share valuable information and resources on social media. By following these accounts and engaging with their content, individuals can stay informed about the latest research, news, and events related to liver cancer prevention. Social media platforms also provide a platform for individuals to share their own experiences and tips for reducing their risk of developing liver cancer.

In conclusion, utilizing online resources for liver cancer prevention can be a powerful tool for individuals who have a higher risk of developing this deadly disease. By accessing reputable medical websites, online support groups, and social media platforms, individuals can educate themselves on the steps they can take to lower their risk. By staying informed, connected, and engaged with these online resources, individuals can empower themselves to take control of their health and reduce their risk of developing liver cancer.

# How To Reduce Liver Cancer Risk

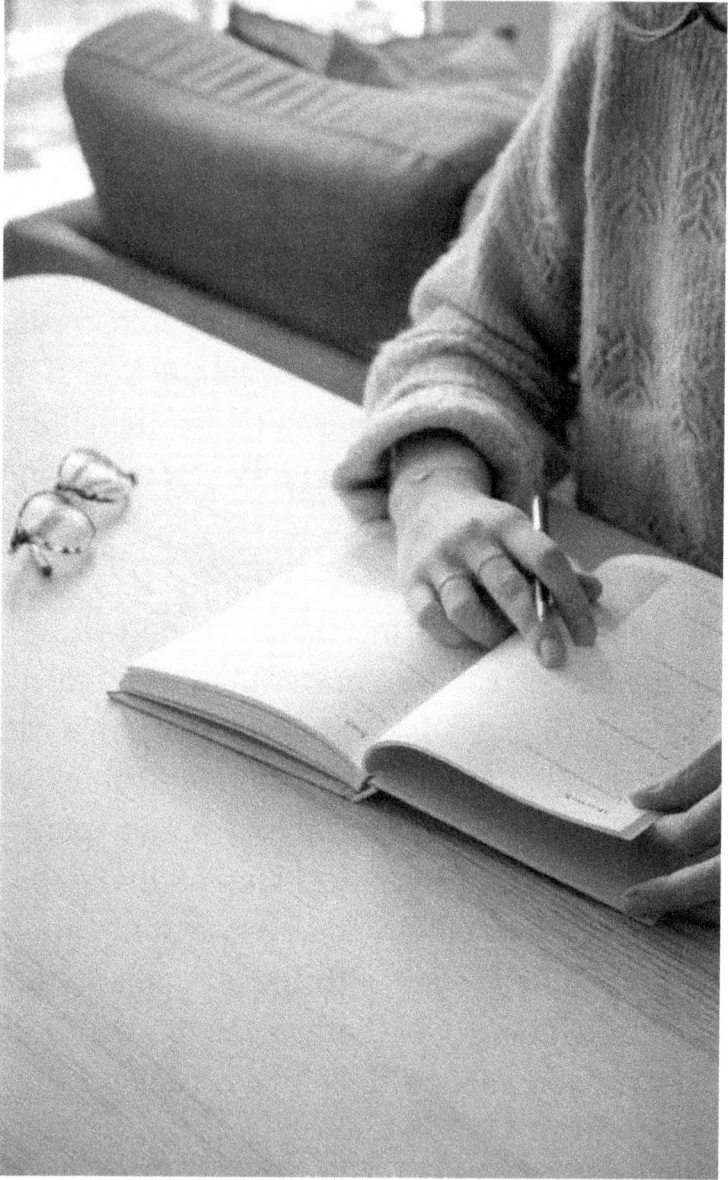

# Chapter 6

# Creating a Personalized Liver Cancer Prevention Plan

## Setting Realistic Goals for Lowering Liver Cancer Risk

Setting realistic goals for lowering your liver cancer risk is essential in maintaining a healthy lifestyle and preventing the development of this serious disease. By implementing specific strategies and making positive changes in your daily routine, you can significantly reduce your risk of developing liver cancer.

One key goal to set when aiming to lower your liver cancer risk is to maintain a healthy weight. Being overweight or obese can increase your risk of developing liver cancer, so it's important to focus on eating a balanced diet and engaging in regular physical activity. Setting a goal to achieve and maintain a healthy weight can have a significant impact on reducing your risk of liver cancer.

Another important goal to consider is limiting your alcohol consumption. Excessive alcohol intake is a major risk factor for liver cancer, so setting a goal to reduce or eliminate alcohol from your diet can greatly reduce your risk.

By setting specific limits on your alcohol consumption and sticking to them, you can take a proactive step towards lowering your risk of developing liver cancer.

In addition to maintaining a healthy weight and limiting alcohol intake, setting a goal to quit smoking can also help lower your liver cancer risk. Smoking is a known risk factor for liver cancer, so quitting smoking can greatly reduce your risk. Setting a goal to quit smoking and seeking support from healthcare professionals can help you successfully achieve this important goal.

Lastly, setting a goal to get regular screenings and check-ups can help detect any potential issues early on and prevent the development of liver cancer.

By staying proactive about your health and getting regular screenings, you can catch any abnormalities or risk factors early and take action to lower your risk of developing liver cancer. Setting realistic goals and taking steps to achieve them can make a significant impact on reducing your liver cancer risk and maintaining a healthy lifestyle.

## Tracking Progress and Making Adjustments

Tracking your progress is crucial when it comes to reducing your risk of liver cancer. By keeping track of your efforts and the changes you are making in your lifestyle, you can better understand what is working and what may need adjustment.

One way to track your progress is by keeping a journal of your daily habits, such as diet, exercise, and alcohol consumption. This will help you see patterns and identify areas where you may need to make changes.

Another way to track your progress is by monitoring your liver health through regular check-ups with your healthcare provider. They can perform tests to assess the health of your liver and provide guidance on how to improve it. By staying on top of your liver health, you can catch any potential issues early and make the necessary adjustments to lower your risk of liver cancer.

Making adjustments to your lifestyle is an important part of reducing your risk of liver cancer. If you find that certain habits or behaviors are increasing your risk, it is important to make changes to decrease that risk.

For example, if you are a heavy drinker, cutting back on alcohol consumption can significantly reduce your risk of developing liver cancer. Similarly, if you have a poor diet high in processed foods and sugar, making healthier choices can help improve your liver health and lower your risk.

In addition to making changes to your diet and lifestyle, it is important to seek support from healthcare professionals and loved ones. They can provide guidance, encouragement, and accountability as you work towards reducing your risk of liver cancer. By forming a strong support system, you can stay motivated and on track to making the necessary adjustments to lower your risk.

In conclusion, tracking your progress and making adjustments are essential steps in reducing your risk of liver cancer. By monitoring your habits, staying on top of your liver health, making necessary lifestyle changes, and seeking support, you can take proactive steps towards lowering your risk.

Remember, it is never too late to make positive changes and improve your overall health. Start today and take control of your liver cancer risk.

## Celebrating Successes and Staying Motivated

Celebrating successes and staying motivated are essential components in the journey to lower your liver cancer risk. It is important to recognize and acknowledge the positive steps you have taken towards prevention. Whether it's adopting a healthier diet, increasing physical activity, or quitting smoking, every small success is worth celebrating. By focusing on the progress you have made, you can stay motivated and continue on the path to reducing your risk of liver cancer.

One way to celebrate your successes is to set specific goals and milestones for yourself. This could be as simple as committing to eating more fruits and vegetables each day or walking for 30 minutes five times a week. By setting achievable goals and tracking your progress, you can see the positive impact of your efforts and stay motivated to continue making healthy choices. Celebrate each milestone you reach, no matter how small, as it signifies your commitment to lowering your liver cancer risk.

Another important aspect of celebrating successes is to share your achievements with others. Whether it's with friends, family, or a support group, sharing your progress can provide encouragement and motivation.

Celebrate your successes with those who support and encourage you on your journey to reducing your liver cancer risk. Their positive reinforcement can help you stay motivated and continue making healthy choices.

In addition to celebrating successes, it is important to stay motivated by reminding yourself of the reasons why you are working towards lowering your liver cancer risk. Whether it's to live a longer, healthier life, or to reduce the burden on your loved ones, keeping your motivations at the forefront of your mind can help you stay focused and committed. Reflect on your reasons for wanting to reduce your risk of liver cancer regularly to stay motivated and on track.

Overall, celebrating successes and staying motivated are crucial components of lowering your liver cancer risk. By setting goals, sharing your achievements, and reminding yourself of your motivations, you can stay on track and continue making healthy choices. Celebrate each small success, no matter how minor, as it signifies your dedication to your health and well-being. Stay motivated and focused on your goals, and you will be well on your way to reducing your risk of liver cancer.

# How To Reduce Liver Cancer Risk

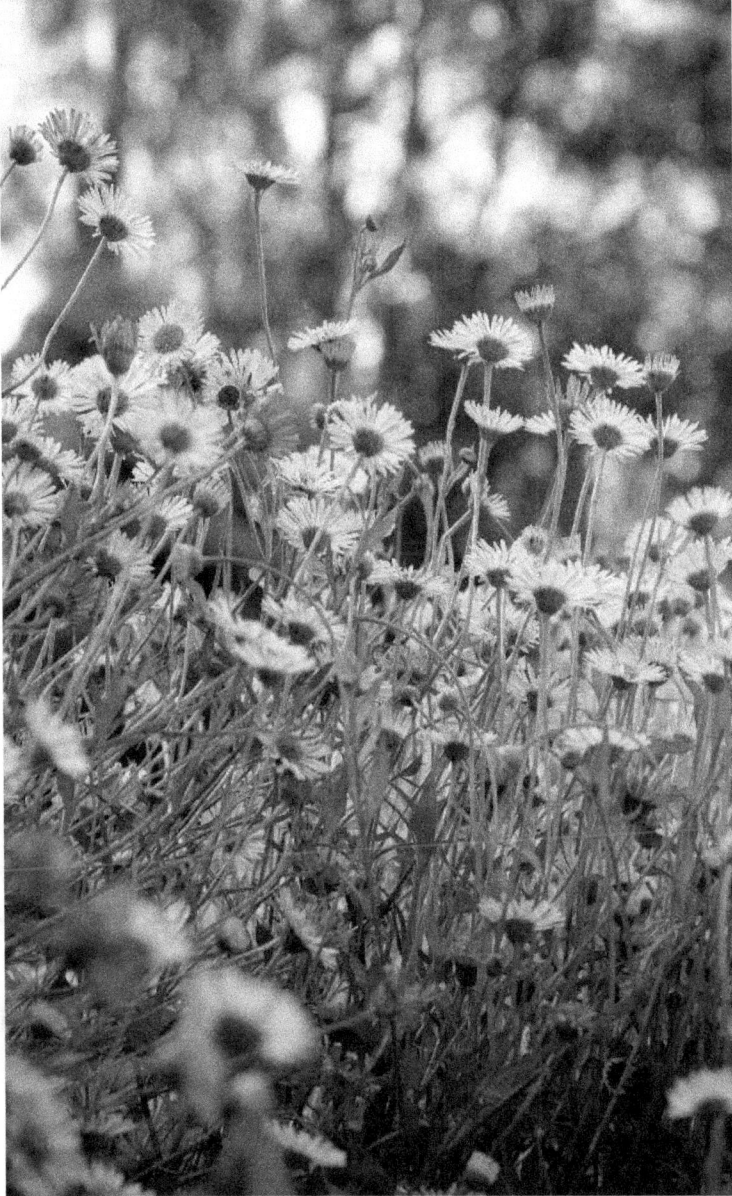

Tips and Strategies for Prevention

# Chapter 7

# Moving Forward with Confidence

## Embracing a Positive Mindset for Liver Cancer Prevention

Embracing a positive mindset is an essential component of lowering your risk for liver cancer. Research has shown that stress and negative emotions can weaken the immune system, making the body more susceptible to developing cancerous cells. By adopting a positive mindset, you can reduce stress levels and boost your overall health, which in turn can help prevent liver cancer from developing.

One way to cultivate a positive mindset is to practice mindfulness and meditation. These practices can help you become more aware of your thoughts and emotions, and can help you develop a more positive and optimistic outlook on life. By taking time each day to focus on the present moment and let go of negative thoughts, you can improve your mental well-being and reduce your risk of developing liver cancer.

Another important aspect of embracing a positive mindset for liver cancer prevention is to focus on self-care and healthy lifestyle habits. This includes eating a balanced diet rich in fruits, vegetables, whole grains, and lean proteins, as well as getting regular exercise and maintaining a healthy weight.

By taking care of your body and making healthy choices, you can reduce inflammation and oxidative stress in the body, both of which are risk factors for liver cancer.

It's also important to surround yourself with positive and supportive people who can help you stay motivated and on track with your health goals. By building a strong support network of friends, family, and healthcare providers, you can stay accountable and encouraged to make positive lifestyle changes that can lower your risk of developing liver cancer.

Remember, you're not alone in this journey, and having a positive support system can make all the difference in your efforts to prevent liver cancer.

In conclusion, embracing a positive mindset is a crucial aspect of lowering your risk for liver cancer. By practicing mindfulness, focusing on self-care and healthy lifestyle habits, and surrounding yourself with positive and supportive people, you can improve your mental and physical well-being and reduce your risk of developing liver cancer.

Remember, a positive outlook and healthy habits can go a long way in protecting your liver health and preventing cancer.

## Continuing Education and Awareness about Liver Cancer

Education is key when it comes to lowering your risk of developing liver cancer. It is important for individuals with risk factors for liver cancer to stay informed about the latest research and recommendations for prevention. By staying up to date on the latest information, you can make informed decisions about your health and take steps to reduce your risk of developing liver cancer.

One important aspect of continuing education about liver cancer is understanding the risk factors associated with the disease. Risk factors for liver cancer include chronic hepatitis B or C infection, heavy alcohol consumption, obesity, and diabetes. By knowing these risk factors, individuals can take steps to address them and lower their risk of developing liver cancer.

In addition to understanding the risk factors for liver cancer, it is important for individuals at risk to be aware of the symptoms of the disease. Symptoms of liver cancer can include unexplained weight loss, abdominal pain, jaundice, and fatigue. By being aware of these symptoms, individuals can seek medical attention if they experience any of them, potentially leading to earlier detection and treatment of the disease.

Another important aspect of continuing education about liver cancer is knowing the screening recommendations for individuals at risk. Screening for liver cancer typically involves imaging tests such as ultrasounds or CT scans, as well as blood tests to check for markers of liver cancer.

By following screening recommendations, individuals at risk can increase their chances of detecting liver cancer at an early, more treatable stage.

Overall, continuing education and awareness about liver cancer are essential for individuals at risk of developing the disease. By staying informed about risk factors, symptoms, and screening recommendations, individuals can take proactive steps to reduce their risk of developing liver cancer and potentially improve their chances of early detection and successful treatment. Remember, knowledge is power when it comes to lowering your liver cancer risk.

## Sharing Knowledge and Tips with Others in the Community

Sharing knowledge and tips with others in the community is a powerful way to help prevent liver cancer and promote overall health and well-being. By sharing your own experiences and insights, you can help others make informed choices about their lifestyle and reduce their risk of developing liver cancer.

In this subchapter, we will explore the importance of sharing knowledge and tips with others in the community, as well as provide some practical strategies for effectively communicating health information to those around you.

One of the most important reasons to share knowledge and tips with others in the community is to raise awareness about the risk factors for liver cancer and the steps that can be taken to lower that risk. Many people are unaware of the factors that can increase their risk of developing liver cancer, such as obesity, excessive alcohol consumption, and chronic viral infections. By sharing information about these risk factors and offering practical tips for reducing them, you can help others take proactive steps to protect their liver health.

Another key reason to share knowledge and tips with others in the community is to provide support and encouragement to those who may be at risk for liver cancer. Dealing with a potentially life-threatening illness can be overwhelming, and having the support of others who understand your situation can make a big difference.

By sharing your own experiences and offering advice and encouragement to others in similar situations, you can help create a strong support network within the community.

When sharing knowledge and tips with others in the community, it is important to communicate in a clear and accessible way. Not everyone may be familiar with medical terminology or complex health concepts, so it is important to use language that is easy to understand and provide practical, actionable advice. By presenting information in a straightforward and relatable manner, you can help ensure that your message is well-received and understood by those you are trying to reach.

In conclusion, sharing knowledge and tips with others in the community is a valuable way to help prevent liver cancer and promote overall health and well-being. By raising awareness, providing support, and communicating effectively, you can empower others to take control of their health and reduce their risk of developing liver cancer. Together, we can work towards a healthier future for ourselves and our community.

# How To Reduce Liver Cancer Risk

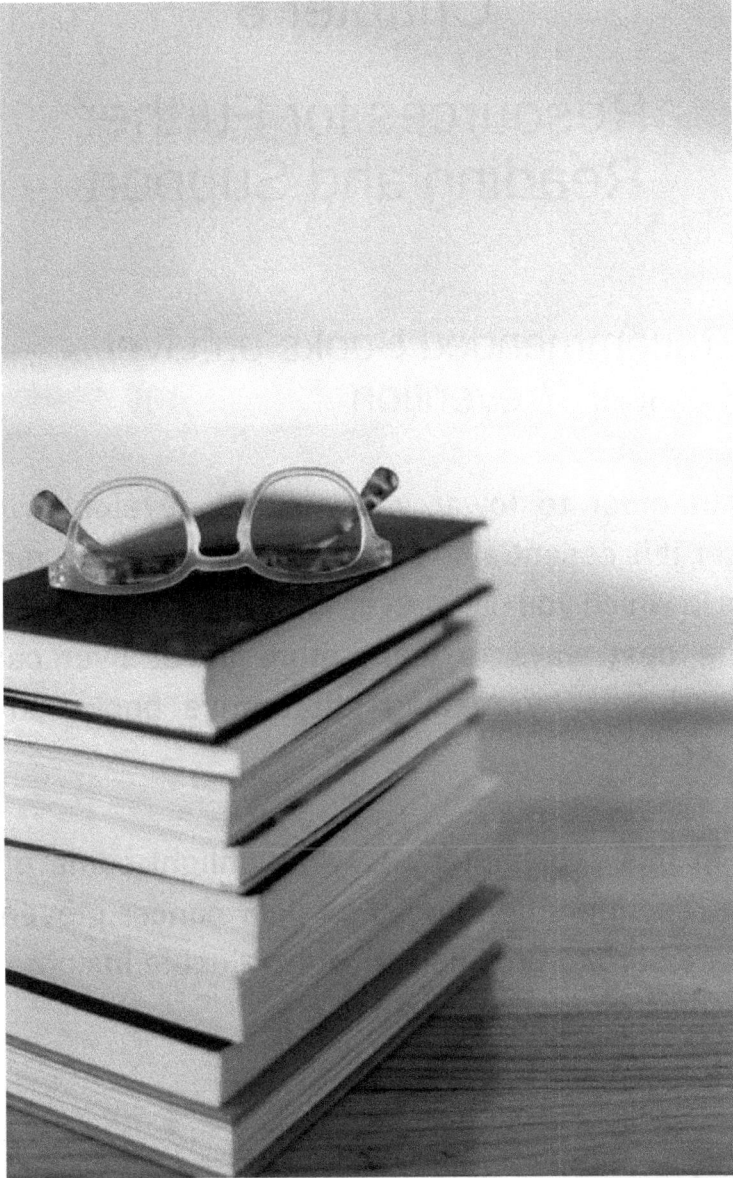

Tips and Strategies for Prevention

# Chapter 8

# Resources for Further Reading and Support

## Recommended Books on Liver Cancer Prevention

In order to lower your risk of developing liver cancer, it is essential to educate yourself on the various ways in which you can prevent this deadly disease. One of the best ways to learn more about liver cancer prevention is by reading informative books on the subject.

In this subchapter, we will highlight some of the most recommended books on liver cancer prevention that are sure to provide you with valuable insights and strategies for reducing your risk.

One highly recommended book on liver cancer prevention is "The Liver Healing Diet" by Dr. Sandra Cabot. This comprehensive guide offers practical tips and advice on how to optimize liver function through diet and lifestyle changes.

By following the recommendations outlined in this book, you can significantly reduce your risk of developing liver cancer and other liver-related diseases.

Another must-read book for those looking to lower their liver cancer risk is "Liver Rescue" by Anthony William. This groundbreaking book delves into the importance of liver health and provides readers with a wealth of information on how to support and protect this vital organ.

By implementing the strategies outlined in this book, you can take proactive steps towards preventing liver cancer and promoting overall well-being.

For those interested in a more holistic approach to liver cancer prevention, "The Liver Cleanse" by Dr. Sandra McRae is an excellent resource. This book offers practical advice on how to detoxify and rejuvenate the liver through natural remedies and lifestyle changes. By incorporating the principles outlined in this book into your daily routine, you can help safeguard your liver against cancer and other diseases.

In addition to these recommended books, there are many other valuable resources available that can help you lower your liver cancer risk. By taking the time to educate yourself on the various strategies for prevention, you can empower yourself to make informed decisions about your health and well-being.

Remember, knowledge is power, and by arming yourself with the information found in these books, you can take proactive steps towards reducing your risk of developing liver cancer.

## Websites and Organizations for Liver Cancer Prevention

One of the most important ways to reduce your risk of developing liver cancer is by staying informed about the latest research and recommendations for prevention. Fortunately, there are many websites and organizations dedicated to providing information and support for individuals at risk of liver cancer. By utilizing these resources, you can stay up to date on the latest developments in prevention strategies and access valuable tools for managing your risk.

One such organization that provides valuable information on liver cancer prevention is the American Liver Foundation. Their website offers a wealth of resources, including information on risk factors, screening recommendations, and lifestyle changes that can help reduce your risk of developing liver cancer. Additionally, the American Liver Foundation offers support groups and educational materials for individuals at risk of liver cancer, providing a valuable network of resources for those seeking to lower their risk.

Another valuable resource for individuals at risk of liver cancer is the Centers for Disease Control and Prevention (CDC) website. The CDC provides information on liver cancer prevention strategies, including vaccination for hepatitis B and C, maintaining a healthy weight, and avoiding excessive alcohol consumption. By visiting the CDC website, you can access evidence-based recommendations for reducing your risk of developing liver cancer and learn more about the latest research in the field.

For individuals looking to connect with others who are at risk of liver cancer, the Cancer Support Community offers a variety of resources and support groups for individuals affected by liver cancer. By joining a support group, you can connect with others who are facing similar challenges and share strategies for reducing your risk of developing liver cancer.

The Cancer Support Community also provides educational materials and resources for individuals seeking to learn more about liver cancer prevention strategies.

In conclusion, staying informed about liver cancer prevention strategies is essential for individuals at risk of developing this disease. By utilizing websites and organizations dedicated to liver cancer prevention, you can access valuable information, resources, and support to help you lower your risk. Whether you are looking for evidence-based recommendations, support groups, or educational materials, there are many resources available to help you in your journey to reduce your risk of developing liver cancer.

## Additional Resources for Individuals at High Risk of Liver Cancer

If you have been identified as being at high risk for liver cancer, there are additional resources available to help you lower your risk and improve your overall health. These resources can provide you with valuable information, support, and guidance to help you on your journey towards reducing your risk of developing liver cancer.

# How To Reduce Liver Cancer Risk

One valuable resource for individuals at high risk of liver cancer is support groups. Joining a support group can provide you with a sense of community and understanding from others who are also at risk. These groups can offer emotional support, practical advice, and a safe space to share your experiences and concerns with others who can relate.

Another important resource for individuals at high risk of liver cancer is access to healthcare professionals who specialize in liver health. Consulting with a liver specialist or hepatologist can provide you with personalized guidance and treatment options to help manage your risk factors and improve your liver health. These professionals can help you develop a personalized plan to lower your risk of developing liver cancer.

Educational resources are also crucial for individuals at high risk of liver cancer. There are many books, websites, and online resources available that can provide you with valuable information on how to reduce your risk of liver cancer. These resources can help you better understand the risk factors, symptoms, and prevention strategies associated with liver cancer.

In addition, lifestyle resources such as nutritionists, exercise specialists, and mental health professionals can also be valuable tools for individuals at high risk of liver cancer. These professionals can help you make positive lifestyle changes, such as improving your diet, increasing physical activity, and managing stress, which can all help reduce your risk of developing liver cancer.

By utilizing these additional resources and seeking support from healthcare professionals, support groups, and educational materials, individuals at high risk of liver cancer can take proactive steps to lower their risk and improve their overall health. Remember, you are not alone in this journey, and there are resources available to help you every step of the way.

# Author Notes & Acknowledgments

First and foremost, I would like to express my deepest gratitude to the people who inspired and supported me throughout the journey of writing this book. This project would not have been possible without their unwavering belief in me and their invaluable contributions.

To my wife, thank you for your constant encouragement and understanding. Your love and support have been my anchor during the challenging times of researching and writing this book. Your belief in my ability to make a difference in people's lives has been my driving force.

I would also like to disclose that this book contains some renewed artificial intelligence-generated content. I really appreciate very recent technological innovation by outstanding scientists and of course our reader's understanding.

Lastly, I want to express my deepest gratitude to the readers of this book. I sincerely hope the strategies and methods outlined within these pages will provide you with the knowledge and tools needed to truly make your life much better. Your commitment to seeking any good solutions and willingness to explore multiple methods is commendable.

# Author Bio

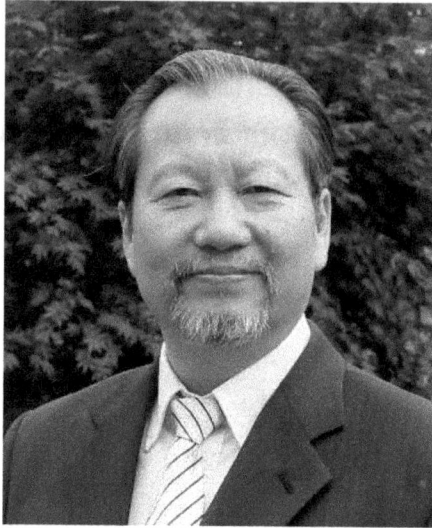

Johnson Wu earned his MD in 1982. With over 40 years of clinical experience, he has worked in hospitals in Zhejiang and Shanghai, China, as well as the Royal Marsden Hospital (part of Imperial College) in London, UK.

Upon the recommendation of Sir Aaron Klug, the president of The Royal Society and a Nobel Prize winner in Chemistry, Dr. Wu was honorably awarded a British Royal Society Fellowship. He has published medical books and articles in seven countries and currently practices medicine in Canada.

www.ingramcontent.com/pod-product-compliance
Lightning Source LLC
Chambersburg PA
CBHW060256030426
42335CB00014B/1718